TO LOVE:

THIS COUPON IS

— good for one —

Breakfast In Bed...

THIS COUPON IS

— good for one —

Dinner And A Movie...

THIS COUPON IS

— good for one —

Night On The Town...

THIS C♥UP♥N IS

— good for one —

A Weekend Getaway...

THIS COUPON IS

— good for one —

Game Night...

THIS COUPON IS

— good for one —

Friday Night Drinks...

THIS C♥UP♥N IS

— good for one —

Just Me And You Time...

THIS COUPON IS

— good for one —

A Sensual Massage...

THIS C♡UP♡N IS

— good for one —

Surprise Me With Flowers...

THIS C♥UP♥N IS

— good for one —

Romantic Dinner...

THIS COUPON IS

— good for one —

Date To The Movies...

THIS C♥UP♥N IS

— good for one —

Half-Hour Massage

THIS COUPON IS

— *good for one* —

Eat Dessert Before Dinner...

THIS COUPON IS

— good for one —

Love Me Like Never Before...

THIS COUPON IS

— good for one —

Serve My Favorite
Meal To Me Naked...

THIS COUPON IS

--- *good for one* ---

Undress Me With Your Teeth...

THIS C♥UP♥N IS

good for one

Morning Sex....

THIS COUPON IS

— good for one —

Quickie...

THIS COUPON IS

— good for one —

A "Yes" Day...

THIS COUPON IS

— *good for one* —

Erotic Movie...

THIS COUPON IS

— good for one —

Get Kisses Anywhere
You Want Them...

THIS COUPON IS

— good for one —

Spend Time Cooking Together...

THIS C♥UP♥N IS

— *good for one* —

Date Night Out For Drinks...

THIS COUPON IS

— good for one —

Getting The Car Washed...

THIS C♥UP♥N IS

good for one

A Relaxing Foot Massage...

THIS COUPON IS

— good for one —

Outdoor Adventure...

THIS COUPON IS

— *good for one* —

Day Of Compliments...

THIS C♥UP♥N IS

— *good for one* —

Car DJ For A Day...

THIS COUPON IS

good for one

Movie Night Out...

THIS C♥UP♥N IS

— good for one —

Personal Bartender...

THIS COUPON IS

— good for one —

Day Of Doing Dishes...

THIS COUPON IS

— good for one —

A Nap With No Interruptions...

THIS COUPON IS

— good for one —

Day At The Beach...

THIS COUPON IS

— good for one —

A Love Letter...

THIS C♡UP♡N IS

S.J. _(signature)_ good for one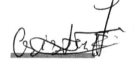

Trying Something Completely New...

THIS COUPON IS

— good for one —

Day In Pajamas...

THIS COUPON IS

— good for one —

A Romantic Dinner For Two...

THIS COUPON IS

— good for one —

A Free Wish...

THIS COUPON IS

— *good for one* —

One Big Bear Hug...

THIS C♥UP♥N IS

— good for one —

Go out dancing...

THIS COUPON IS

_____ good for one _____

S.J. [signature]

Shower Together

THIS COUPON IS

— good for one —

THIS COUPON IS

— good for one —

THIS COUPON IS

— *good for one* —

THIS COUPON IS

— good for one —

Printed in Great Britain
by Amazon